Fit After 40

Everything You Need to Know to Look Young, Feel Young and Stay Young at Any Age

Sarah Tyler

Copyright

Terms of Use

Any information provided in this book is through the author's interpretation. The author has done strenuous work to reassure the accuracy of this subject. If you wish you attempt any of the practices provided in this book, you are doing so with your own responsibility. The author will not be held accountable for any misinterpretations or misrepresentations of the information provided here.

All information provided is done so with every effort to represent the subject, but does not guarantee that your life will change. The author shall not be held liable for any direct or indirect damages that result from reading this book.

Contents

Introduction

So by now you've reached a successful point of your life. By now you've gotten to the point where you need to relax yourself and stop working so hard all the time. Well, not really but you kind of get the point.

Anyways, the fact that you're reading this book is because you're curious or you want to know about how to stay fit after 40, give or take the numbers of how old you are.

Either way, you want to know how to lose weight and stay healthy at the same time. Even if you don't need to lose weight this book will tell you how to maintain a healthy body so it works just as well.

The whole point of staying fit is the fact that you chose to stay fit. I don't know how many times I can literally emphasize this to you, but you have to know it.

Everything that you do in life is by your own choice and no one else. Even if something bad happens to you then it's probably something that was influenced by the choices that you've made.

The whole "being at the wrong place at the wrong time" can also apply because you chose to be at a specific location at a specific time. It is by your own choice and no one else's.

Of course, people can influence you to a certain point but in the end, you are going to be the one making the decisions.

Therefore, if you just suddenly decide that dieting and staying healthy isn't going to work for you then it's not going to work for you.

However, if you believe that dieting and staying healthy will work for you and that you can do it then you'll be able to achieve your goal.

Now I'm not saying that the plan that I'm going to lay out for you is going to help you 100%. You have to realize that everyone is different and everyone has different needs.

This book is written so you can get a clue as to what you should do. If you want to go into more of a detailed description of what you should do then that's something that you have to do on your spare time with a professional.

By no excuse should you not decide to stay healthy. Understand that being healthy does not always mean being skinny.

Being skinny is a different matter and everyone has their own view of how thin you must be to be considered skinny. Though, you should always choose to live healthy rather than skinny.

Think about it, skinny and healthy can be the same or it cannot be the same.

If you're skinny and healthy then that's a good accomplishment for you and I have no idea why you are reading this book unless if you're trying to maintain that balance.

If you're skinny but not healthy then that's not the way to go. If you're healthy and not skinny then there's something wrong. Most likely, if you're healthy then you should also be skinny.

It's like a bonus for your body. Plus, when you're healthy your body will be toned. Take this quote into consideration:

"Being skinny makes you look better with clothes on. Being healthy and fit makes you look better with clothes off."

I know that sounds sort of sexual but, hey, we all have insecurities about our bodies so let that be a motivating factor for you to tone your body up. Besides, being fit will allow you to appreciate losing weight compared to being thin.

If you're losing weight just to be thin then you're not going to feel as great as someone who is losing weight to be fit. Being fit and being thin is an everyday choice.

You might as well just chose to be fit so you can feel healthy and confident about the body that you're trying to achieve.

You should also realize that when you chose to go on a diet you are choosing a life long program that you should not stray away from.

It's going to take months and years to get the body that you want and even then you will have to spend the rest of your life trying to maintain that body.

I know it sounds hard but it really isn't. Dieting is achievable with dedication and patience. If you set out your goals and you stick by them then you'll be on the right track to success.

Chapter 1 – Dieting

So this chapter is going to give you the layout of what dieting is and why you would need to diet.

There are plenty of reasons as to why you should go on a diet compared to the questions of why you should not go on a diet. Well, the ironic part about dieting is the fact that it has the word die in it.

Of course, if you're dieting the wrong way then you might possibly die from it. It's a possibility but don't quote me on that.

Anyways, this chapter is mainly just a little breakdown about what you should do and what you should not do when you are starting the diet plan.

They're good tips to keep in mind and it won't hurt you to remember some of them as they will come in handy in the future.

Gaining Weight

No one enjoys the fact that they have to be careful about their weight. Nobody enjoys the fact that we have to gain weight.

No one wants to bother themselves into losing weight. Unfortunately, we have to watch our weight and we have to lose weight if we are overweight.

It is part of life and we will just have to deal with it. It's going to be a hard process for some people in the beginning but it will become a habit once you keep going.

You should know that gaining weight doesn't happen overnight. It happens through time.

All those junk foods that you ate during those previous months of partying and feasting, all those sodas, all those chips, all those cakes, and all those unhealthy snacks that you ate when you were hungry has accumulated into your weight.

Sure, there might have been some occasional times when you've worked out at the gym or took a jog around the park, but did you ever ask yourself how much you've ate and how much you've burned off? Probably not and that's probably why you've gained weight.

A good amount of calorie intake for an average person is about 1,200 calories per day. From there, you give or take some calories depending on how fast or how slow your metabolism is.

However, if you end up eating more calories than what your body needs then your body will end up turning those excessive calories into fat. This is one reason as to how you gain weight.

Another reason can be your genes. Your genes don't play as high of a role in gaining weight but it's the starting point. If your family has a linage of low metabolism then you will be born with low metabolism.

This is more of a luck factor as some people are born with high metabolism. However, you are able to change the rate of your metabolism on your own and that is through exercising, which brings me into another point.

It doesn't matter how healthy you eat as a person. If you do not exercise then you cannot lose weight. Well, you can but only to a certain extent.

It's actually recommended that you exercise anyways, especially for the benefits that you get through exercising. Plus, you'll feel great both inside and outside.

The Pitfalls of Dieting

Why do we need to diet? Yes, it might require a lot of efforts and yes it might be frustrating sometimes because you have to cut back on the foods that you would normally eat; however, the results will be worth it and your body will be the proof of that.

Of course, not all diet plans are going to work for you. It's always recommended that you see a professional before thinking up a plan for yourself.

I mean, if you know what you are doing then there is no problem, but if you are unsure as to how you should approach your diet plan then a professional is the way to go.

Nevertheless, everyone has their own thoughts about what dieting is. For most people, they think dieting is a process that will help you lose weight quickly and efficiently.

That is not the case. Dieting is a long process and just like how it takes years for you to gain weight, dieting will take years for you to get rid of that weight. Even so, there are a few dieting pitfalls that most people land themselves into.

For one thing, it's the so called fad diet. I'm unsure if this trend is still going around as commonly as the others but it's still here.

The fad diet is a dieting program that requires you to remove a food group from your daily eating habits.

You're probably wondering why that's not a good idea, especially if they are getting rid unhealthy food.

Technically, the fad diet is when you get rid of something that you should eat rather than what you not eat.

It also includes the unusual mixtures of drinking ingredients, which is also not good because if you're not mixing the proper ingredients then there is something bad that is going to happen to you later on in the long run.

Also, during the process of the fad diet, you will start to feel less energetic then before. That's because your energy is slowly draining from you due to lack of nutrients and the diet becomes a lot worse in the long run because once you stop, you'll be gaining back the weight that you were trying so hard to lose.

The second pitfall of dieting is the calories. Now, we all know that calories are important to keep track of during the dieting process.

This way, you won't start to over eat and you'll know exactly how much calories you're taking in. However, when most people do not bother to follow a steady diet plan and try to calculate the amount of calories that they are eating everyday, they will become frustrated. It's expected.

Trying to remember every calorie that you take in and counting them all by the end of the day is going to seem very troublesome for you after a week or so. It's going to make you want to give up before trying the actual diet.

The third pitfall of dieting is the food. This goes hand in hand with the fad diet and the calories diet.

When most people want to lose weight their first choice is to eat less. Thus, the fad diet is placed in position because they are getting rid of certain foods that they should eat to stay healthy.

When people plan to eat less, they choose to pay attention to the calories that they eat. Thus, the calorie intake diet is placed in position.

Also, when people eat less than what they are supposed to, they will start to crave. They will eat the food that they want and if it's high in calories then they will try to starve themselves for the rest of the day.

This is bad because, one, they will feel hungry and uncomfortable due to the fact that their bodies do not have the proper nutrients that they need. Two, instead of losing fat, they will start to lose muscle and gain more fat in the process.

Despite these pitfalls of dieting, it does not mean that dieting doesn't have benefits. As I've mentioned before, dieting has a lot of benefits.

Of course, that's only if you're doing it right. These pitfalls that I've mentioned are only a glimpse of what to not do during a diet.

If you want a more detailed explanation of what not to do then you should skip to the Do's and Don'ts chapter.

How it Works

The way dieting works is very tricky. Many people want to lose weight at a quick rate, but that's not going to work out when you are "dieting".

This is because dieting is a process that will take months or years to accomplish depending on your current weight and the weight that you're trying to achieve.

Now, you're probably thinking in the back of your mind about how other people are able to lose their weight in a short amount of time. Newsflash, it's going to backfire.

When you lose weight within a short amount of time, the weight that you've lost is going to come right back as soon as you stop the program that you were doing.

It's going to be worse because you'll most likely gain more weight in the process and it'll be harder for you to lose that weight again.

The best method of dieting is slow and steady. No matter what dieting method you use, you're going to need discipline and determination.

So instead of using your double Ds on a method that's not going to greatly benefit you, use it on a method that will keep you healthy and fit for the rest of your life.

Of course, dieting doesn't necessarily mean that you can only eat just fruits and vegetables.

You're kind of leaning towards the vegetarian aspect of dieting when you think like that. Of course, even vegetarians eat different varieties of food besides vegetables.

How do I know? I've had my fair share of vegetarian food seeing as my mother is a vegetarian herself.

Anyways, the way dieting works is actually very simple. All you have to do and I've probably mentioned this already, is take in the amount of calories that your body actually needs and exercise the amount of calories that you've eaten. It's simple, it's easy, and it'll make you feel healthy.

Do's and Don'ts

These are the typical, but important, do's and don'ts of dieting.

Though, rather than focusing on the don'ts, which I've already mentioned some earlier before, I'll focus more on the do's.

I'll start with the don'ts because these are more important to keep in mind only because if you remember what you should not do, it's easier to think about what's the proper thing to do. Anyways, things you should not do:

1. Starving:

Starving is very, if not immensely, common for people to do when they want to lose weight. I don't know why. I have never known why and I could never understand why. I honestly love food and I could never picture starving myself in order to lose weight because I won't be able to resist my hunger.

Even so, you're actually gaining weight if you try to starve yourself. That's because your body doesn't know that you want to lose weight. All it knows is the fact that you are starving and in order to preserve your energy, your body will convert your muscles into fat.

Thus, you will be gaining more weight than before. In addition, your metabolism will be lowered so it'll take longer for you to digest your food. Not only that but you will also be more vulnerable to other diseases that can endanger your life. If anything, you might be diagnosed with anorexia.

2. Vomiting:

This is almost the same as starving, but worse. There's actually no point in eating if you are going to throw up everything that you've just eaten. Though, I'm not supporting the idea of starving but this method is also dangerous and harmful to your body.

In the beginning, when you start to vomit the food that you've eaten, you'll notice that nothing is wrong. This is because you are still in the beginning stages of method.

Later on, you'll start noticing a slight change to your body. You'll start feeling sick and sluggish and if you keep going, you might even take the first step to having eating disorders.

3. Exercising:

Now I know I've mentioned a little bit about how exercise is good for you. Exercising is very good for you and is actually recommended my many doctors or any health professionals.

However, even if exercising is good for your health and body, it is good to an extent. That means that you shouldn't overdo it.

A good daily workout is about 30 minutes to an hour depending on how intense your workout is. Doing an intense workout for more than an hour can cause harm to your body over time whether you realize it or not. It doesn't matter how strong you think your body is. Just put a limit as to how much exercise you do all at once.

4. Pills:

In the present day society advertisement is everything. If your advertisement sounds legitimate enough to get your viewers to order from you then you are doing a wonderful job of making business.

Unfortunately, as a viewer, you cannot believe everything that you hear on TV. Actually, there are scams everywhere so you really cannot believe everything that you hear or read or see, period.

This is a very good life lesson for anyone who has not yet done so: research what you don't know or what seems too good to be true.

Many industries have already mass produced weight loss pills for the market to sell. These weight loss pills are made for the purpose of losing weight at a fast rate and/or without you trying to lose weight.

Does this sound too good to be true? It does! That's because it's not true. Majority of the time, these weight loss pills that you're buying doesn't even do what it's supposed to do.

Rather, it does the opposite. There are even a few types of labeling involved that the industries put on just to get you to believe them. The ones that I'm about to list are the common ones that almost everyone should have stumbled across by now.

All Natural Ingredients:

Natural ingredients are always the best because it's natural. It's produced straight from Mother Nature. It isn't filled with chemicals and it isn't artificially made with ingredients that you've never heard of before.

However, just because the labeling says natural ingredients don't mean that the ingredients are at all natural. I'm pretty sure that if you were to take a look at the ingredients, you would find nothing natural about it.

You'd probably find words that you've never seen before, or words that you are unable to pronounce. Obviously, if you can't pronounce an ingredient then there is nothing natural about it and there's not much that you can do about it.

The companies are free to place their products on the market as long as it is not approved from the FDA that it is harmful.

Scientifically Proven:

I know that this might be a hard one to tell whether it's trying to cheat you out of your money or not, but there's a way.

Notice how it says scientifically proven without giving you any additional information about how it was proven or who approved it. Basically, it's a labeling that can easily cheat you into buying it.

When this happens you are expected to do some research. If you are too lazy to do a quick five minute research of the product that you are planning to buy then don't buy it. Chances are, it's not good for you and chances are, it's going to waste your money.

Government Approved:

Understand that the government does not approve everything. The government already has a lot of issues that they have to deal with for the people.

They do not have the time to approve everything that is on demand. Even if they did approve everything, it isn't as if that everything is going to be approved properly.

For those of you who have your own ideas about what the government does, you should have an idea that they couldn't care less about what products are being sold on the market and how harmful it could be to you. They have other people to take care of those issues for them.

Now, here are the things that you should do:

Seek advice

When we start on something new that we don't have any idea with, we want advice. However, we don't just want anyone's advice; we want advice from a professional or someone who has experience on the topic that we are seeking help on. This way, it'll stop us from making poor choices along the way.

There are a lot of people that you can approach when you want advice about how to stay healthy.

Many people would normally confront a doctor for help, but doctors can only tell you the vague idea of how to be healthy. Their job is to make you healthy again, not tell you how to stay healthy.

There are a few common professionals that you should approach if you want a more detailed explanation of how to stay healthy, some of which is what I've listed down below.

Dieticians:

These professionals should be on the top of your list when you are about to engage yourself in the dieting process.

Dieticians are licensed professionals that are paid to help you with your needs. They have a wide range of knowledge about what you should do to in order to lose weight and what you should not do.

You'll probably have to go through a physical check up before they can decide what type of dieting plan you should engage yourself in, but don't quote me on that.

Usually, when consulting a dietician, they will normally tell you the right amount of calories that you can consume without eating too much or too little.

Take note of everything that they tell you because it is important for you to know what you will be doing later on.

Physical Trainers:

If you want a physical trainer then it's going to be expected that you will have to do majority of your physical training in the gym. Either that or you can hire a private physical trainer, but I believe that they are more costly.

Though, physical trainers are good to have around. These are the type of people who are paid to make sure that you are doing the proper training in order to meet your goals.

They will make up a plan that will fit you the most and they will give you both cardio and strength based exercises to follow throughout your training.

I greatly recommend that you have a physical trainer to help you, especially when you don't have a busy schedule on your hand. Plus, physical trainers tend to be flexible with your time schedule, at least most are. Even if you don't get to have the chance to meet with them very often, most physical trainers will give you a training program to do on your own when they are not around to guide you.

Therapists:

Now, you're probably thinking why you would consult with a therapist. Truth is, you don't necessarily have to, but for the people who tend to closely tie up foods and feelings, you should.

If you ever noticed yourself eating unhealthy snacks when you are feeling sad or depressed then you know that you need to go see a therapist.

In life, you are going to be sad many times. If you eat when you are sad then that's one pound gained for every tear drop that rolls down your eyes.

That one pound is going to then accumulate and you're going to end up being overweight. If you've noticed this trend for a long time now then you need to find help immediately.

Do not spend your time waiting because it will get worse. I cannot tell you what your therapist might tell you because I'm sure that it's different with everyone.

Most likely, she will recommend you to a dietician in order to help you lose the weight that you've gained.

The Plan

Having the proper diet plan that fits your needs are of absolute importance. Not every diet plan works for the same people.

If you've had a diet plan that was closely similar to someone and you noticed that the plan worked for them but not for you then you should know why.

Your diet plan might be similar to someone and it might not. It all depends on your body and on your activity rate.

Normally, you would eat about 1,200 calories per day in order for your body to completely digest everything without having to store the excessive food as fat. However, that normal balance is only an estimate of an average person.

If you are less active then the average person then you need to cut down that 1,200. If you are more active then the average person then you need to add more calories to that 1,200. In the end, it depends on you.

You should know how active you are. Of course, if you are doing this on your own without any professional help, it's always good to start small.

If you need to cut down the amount of calories that you should take in then cut down 100 calories. If you noticed that you're still gaining some weight then decrease another 100. If you see that you've remained the same weight as before then decrease another 100 and stop there.

The same applies if you are adding more calories. Remember, you want to eat a good amount that will allow your body to cut down about one to two pounds per week.

I know that it seems very little but if you want the healthiest results then you just have to accept it. Plus, the weight that you've lost is less likely to come back if you were to take a short break from dieting.

When choosing a plan for yourself, you want to make sure that it is easy for you to continue that plan.

Obviously, you are not going to make a plan for yourself to cut back on food and expect yourself to follow through it immediately. Even if you do, you are not going to last for a very long time.

Always have some sort of realistic expectations for yourself when making your own plans. The amount of time it will take for you to lose weight will depend on how much weight you want to lose.

Still, you should not let that fact discourage you. I know you want to lose weight fast but even when you've lost the weight that you've wanted to lose you will have to learn how to maintain it. Either way, you have to take it slow and steady.

Remember, losing one to two pounds a week is healthy. If you lose about three to four pounds a week then that's fine too, but you'll need to slow down if you start going over that amount.

If anything, I recommend that you consult a specialist if you are not sure of what you are doing.

Make sure to always, always, always do research before heading off to something, especially when it includes your health.

Even if you think you know what you are doing, research anyways to be 100% sure. It wouldn't hurt to spend that extra five minutes of your life gaining knowledge that could benefit you.

Never bother yourself with plans that want you to cut off certain foods unless if you are cutting off unhealthy junk food. Never bother with plans that require you to take any type of pills to lose weight. Like I've mentioned before, it is not healthy and can damage your body.

Keep in mind that you should already know what your daily schedule is. When you start your diet plan, start planning out your weekly schedule. It will help you stay on task and you won't have to stress out about missing a workout time.

It's good to know that you can trust yourself but it's even better if you can write your schedule down on paper or your phone.

The plan has to fit your schedule. If you are the type of person who works all day for five days a week then its best if you plan your workout days during the weekends.

If you end up doing everything on a whim then not only will your schedule be inconsistent but you might just end up giving up on the program altogether.

In addition to that, you can confuse your body with your inconsistency so you will end up making it harder for yourself to lose weight.

This is why scheduling is important. Plus, it shouldn't take you more than five minutes to plan for the week either and you'll be more organized if you do.

You'll find that it's also more convenient for you to maintain a schedule simply because you will follow it more often. Of course, even when keeping a schedule, make sure that the time between each schedule is reasonable.

Give yourself a short 5 minute break in between each new event that you have to finish. I recommend writing everything on your phone because it's harder to lose.

Also, in the case where you end up being off schedule, you can record your mistakes for future purposes.

No one enjoy making mistakes so by the fact that you can see what you did wrong should be enough for you to want to correct it the next time.

Once you get into the habit of scheduling everything you'll find that your life will be a lot simpler than before. Not to mention that you'll be less stressed in life.

A Successful Diet Plan

In order to have a successful diet plan, you need to plan. As I've mentioned before, having a schedule is crucial and very important when you start dieting.

If you have always been a natural planner then this is easy for you. If you this will be your first time then play around to see what planning method works best for you.

I personally like to plan my schedule with my phone. It's easy because I take my phone everywhere with me.

Though, I also own a small white board that I use to list any important dates or any upcoming events. It works just fine for me because my phone is non-existent when I am at home.

A diet plan does not only include planning for the future, but it includes recording the past. If you have tried many dieting programs in the past you should've kept a separate journal for each program that you've tried.

This is important because it'll allow you to look back at what you did. You'll be able to see what worked and what didn't.

By using your past achievements and mistakes, you are able to make a proper diet plan that will completely fit you. If you've never kept a journal of your previous records or if this is your first dieting program, start making a journal of your progress.

It doesn't even have to be on paper. You can even use Microsoft Excel to help you keep your records in check.

The reason why I mentioned Microsoft Excel is because I think that it's the best program you can use to keep any long records of data in.

You can even print out the sheets after the page is filled and stuff it in a binder or a folder. It's the same amount of work as using a regular journal.

The only difference is that you are wasting ink. Preferably, I would rather choose a journal simply because I can carry it around with me at all times.

Using a smart phone works too but if you do then I recommend that you use an app called Evernote. It's easy to use and in the case if something were to happen to your phone, you won't lose any data because it's stored online.

It's perfectly fine if you are not sure of what piece of information you should record during your diet program, or how you would record it.

Always remember to put the date down because the date is crucial. You don't necessarily have to note the time you ate, but it'll allow you to know the time gap between each of your snack/meal time.

If you note the time then it'll be easier for you to note the amount of calories you ate during that time.

By the end of the day, make sure you calculate your total amount of calorie consumption. If you start to crave, which will most definitely happen during the dieting period, then you have to get right back on track as soon as you can.

Just because you start craving for one day doesn't mean that you get the rest of the day off. The only exception to that rule is if you craved during your last meal.

At any rate, if you want to see results then looking at yourself in the mirror after a week isn't going to show you much.

You most likely won't notice a change in your figure until after the third week or so. That doesn't mean that you aren't losing weight.

If you want to see the results of your effort then you should weight yourself before the start of each week, or you can measure yourself.

Weights are easier to do because all you need is a scale, but if you are going to measure yourself then its best if you go into details with it. Don't just measure your waist.

Measure your thighs and your arms. When you're done measuring, record it. At the end of each week, measure yourself again.

Repeat the process and sooner or later, you'll start noticing a change in your weight and your body structure.

Remember, start taking about 30 minutes to an hour walk everyday. You might think walking might not do much but it does something and something is always better than nothing.

Think about it. Walking is the easiest exercise that you can do and the fact that you can burn calories just by walking is absolutely amazing. This exercise is especially good for the elderly.

When you walk outside, it's always best to walk around a park or somewhere quiet. Pick a non-polluted area to walk around.

Not only will you be able to breathe in fresh air but you'll be healthy. I recommend walking in the early morning, sometime between 6-8 A.M.

That's because most people are barely heading off to work around 8 in the morning and hardly anyone is up around 6.

Chapter 2 – Exercising

Exercise is important. We need it because our body needs it. It keeps us active and healthy and best of all, it helps us lose weight. However, most people don't enjoy the thought of exercising. Why?

Because when most people think of exercising, they think about the regular workouts at the gym.

They think about that heavy duty, intense workout that leaves you exhausted after half an hour. Well, that's to be expected. However, there are also different types of workout that doesn't leave you completely exhausted.

As I've mentioned before, walking is one option. Of course, if you feel exhausted after doing a short workout at the gym then you know that you need to be fit.

Depending on the type of person you are, you'll feel different after a workout. For me, I feel more focused in my work after doing an intense workout. I don't know if that works for anyone, but from the people I know, it hasn't.

Anyways, don't bother making those common New Year's resolution if you want to lose weight. Saying that you will do something is completely different then actually doing it.

There are actually a lot of excuses that most people will and can make in order to avoid having to exercise. Trust me; if you really wanted to do something then you will do it.

Human determination is powerful if you are determined enough. The one reason that I can understand for anyone is if you were busy.

It's understandable if you cannot fit exercise into your schedule because as a working adult, your work is important.

However, your health is also important. If you are using the excuse of lack of time then you should figure out what your actual schedule is because I'm sure that you cannot work every single hour of your life for all seven days.

Though, it is understandable if you are too tired to start a workout after working so hard for the week, but like I said, walking is also an exercise.

Instead of using the car all the time and spending gas money, walk and bus. I know that some people shiver at the thought of public transportation because, you know, it's public transportation.

However, you should at least take it as an experience that you might need for future purposes, especially if something happens to your car and you don't have a bike.

Another excuse would be that exercise is too boring. I agree. Exercising is boring. You're working out alone. You're sweaty. You're tired. You're dehydrated.

Well, you also choose to make exercise boring. If you want exercise to me more then join a small sports team. I'm sure that there is a bunch of community sports team all around. Either that or you can make up one your own for fun.

Exercise is always more fun in a group then alone. Another option is to multitask. If you still watch TV during your spare time then while you are watching TV, you should use that time to exercise.

For instance, during a commercial you can do ten quick push-ups. Then, for the next commercial, you can do ten quick squats. You can continue this until the show is over.

Not only will you get the exercise you need but you'll also have something to do during a boring commercial rather than just sit there and wait.

Here is the biggest dilemma to exercising: lack of motivation. I'm pretty sure that no one will want to exercise if they do not have the motivation to exercise.

People like immediate results and if they know that they won't get immediate results, the motivation is going to be dead and wiped out from their mind.

It's expected, but you have to change it. I know that the first step into exercising is hard because you have to motivate yourself to actually start the workout. Once you're in the workout, everything will flow together until you decide to stop.

Even if you don't want to take the first step, you have to force yourself to. Man up and do it because no one is going to bother forcing you if you aren't going to budge on your own.

When you start exercising, it's going to become a habit for you after some time. If you're wondering when the best time to exercise during the day is then I would recommend the morning.

I've already mentioned why you should exercise in the morning in the previous chapter, but it's also because you haven't eaten anything yet.

I hope you haven't eaten anything yet before you exercise in the morning. Even so, this is still risky for some people.

Do not immediately eat after you exercise. Sure, you might be tired and exhausted but that's enough of a reason to not eat.

Once you are done exercising, take a short 20-30 minute break before you start to eat.

If you eat immediately after a workout then you will have a higher chance of gaining weight. Thus, the workout that you've just done was basically pointless.

If you are going to workout after you eat then wait for about at least 2-3 hours before working out. This is because you want to fully make sure that your food has completely digested before you start any intense workout for the day.

Types

There are about three different types of exercises that you can do when you start working out. It's always good to have an equal balance of all three of these once you start your workout.

There are plenty of different techniques for each type so you can mix and match however you want, but I recommend that you consult a professional just in case.

The best method I can tell you is to do a different type of exercise once every two weeks. So for about two weeks you'll focus on a certain type, say bone and muscle strength, and for the other two weeks you'll move onto another type, say flexibility.

Make sure that you balance the workout to fit your needs. Even if you think you can do it, it's best if you don't try to push your limit because you can end up hurting yourself in the process.

Just as I've mentioned, one type of exercise is flexibility. Flexibility is pretty simple. It's kind of like Gymnastics but not as intense unless if you wanted it to be. I supposed that a good example would be like yoga.

If you don't know what yoga is, it's basically a series of workout that help improve your flexibility.

I highly recommend that you start doing yoga training, or any other type of training that helps you improve your flexibility. It'll help you a lot in the future when you are older than what you are now.

Flexibility is actually quite useful in your everyday life. If you've noticed a certain pain in your body after a certain pose that you did then you know that your body is not flexible enough.

If you train your flexibility, you'll be able to easily cope with more difficult poses that can help you get through your daily life.

Plus, training your flexibility doesn't take a long amount of time. Anytime will do and you can train almost anywhere.

Usually, if you do any intense poses then you'll only need to spend about 10-15 minutes of your time per day. For any basic pose, just do the regular arm and leg stretch that takes less than one minute for each pose.

Another type of exercise is the cardiovascular type of exercise. This type of workout mainly improves the functions of your lungs.

Usually, those with heart problems would do these types of exercises because it can greatly decrease their chances of getting a heart attack.

These exercises would be more time consuming and can become very intense. Running falls into this category, but there are plenty more.

For the best results, I recommend that you seek advice from a personal trainer before doing any type of exercises from this category.

The last type of exercise would be the bone and muscle strength type. You can consider these exercises to be like a type of body building exercises. Yes, it does include weight lifting and the workout can become very intense.

You can actually do these types of exercises on your own, assuming that you don't overdo your limit. For these types of exercises, a good half an hour is enough for the day. You can boost it to a full hour but if you do that then I would recommend every two days. Because weight lifting can become very intense, it's always good to leave a gap between the workout days.

Chapter 3 – Maintenance

If you think that losing weight is going to be hard then you're going to have a difficult time trying to maintain your weight. Well, not really. Maintaining and losing weight uses practically the same method.

As long as you continue what you were doing before, assuming that it was healthy, then you'll be fine with maintaining your weight.

Though I've mentioned a fair share of tips on how to lose weight, I'll mention them again for the maintenance purposes. Also, it'll be like a little review from what you've just read.

Meal Time

Meal time is fun time. It's when you get to fill up your belly with delicious food that you've either made on your own or bought with your hard earned money. You should always embrace meal time and never ignore them.

You can think of meal time as your child. You can't ignore them because if you do, that's bad for you and your child. Anyways, don't ever skip out on meal time.

Once you start skipping meal time, your body will immediately believe that you are starving and it will start storing your body with fat that was normally your muscle.

You don't want to lose muscle and gain fat. Fats weight more than muscles. Plus, even forcing yourself to skip a meal time will be trouble for you later on because you'll feel the need to overeat in order to fill up your hunger.

When you eat, eat a variety of foods that does not include unhealthy junk foods. Even when eating healthy, it's good to eat a variety of healthy food. It's not good to eat the same type of food all the time.

Your body needs to experience different type of nutrients in order for it to function properly. There are a lot of different varieties of healthy food.

You don't have to eat those that you don't particularly like but make sure you eat a different type every so often to keep your body healthy.

A good amount to eat per day would be five to six meals per day. It not only keeps your metabolism up but it also keeps you full.

It'll stop you from every feeling hungry and there will be less of a chance that you might overeat. You're probably thinking why you should eat five to six meals per day. I know it's a big amount.

However, just because I said five to six meals doesn't mean that they are all main meals. Of course, you already have your three main meals of the day: breakfast, lunch, and dinner.

For the other two or three meals, those will be your snack time. It's easier to keep a balance of five meals per day because the two extras would be brunch (between breakfast and lunch) and linner (between lunch and dinner).

Fitting a sixth meal in will be entirely up to you. Remember to eat a salad or a type of fruit during snack time. They are nutritious, healthy, and fill you up just right.

Exercise

You know the whole idea now. Exercise, exercise, and exercise. Don't overdo your workouts, especially when it is too intense for your body. Going the extra mile is always good but not when it can damage your health.

Exercising is sort of like eating. You have to change your exercise routine every once in a while. It doesn't have to be every week, but at least change it twice a month. That's because your body will start to adapt to the workout that you are doing.

Once your body remembers your exercise routine, it'll be harder for you to lose weight with that routine. That's why it's always best to change it up every so often. It'll make it harder for your body to adjust. Also, don't slack off. If you missed a day of exercise then that is fine because you probably have something to do.

However, don't continue to believe that it will be fine and don't continue to keep putting it off. The longer you put off the need to exercise the harder it will be for you to start again.

Sleep

Sleep is important if you want to stay healthy. You've probably heard your doctor mentioning it many times to you before. If you haven't taken his advice yet then I suggest you start doing so.

Everyone needs about an average amount of eight hours of sleep everyday. You don't necessarily have to reach the eight hour amount.

Six or seven is also good, but eight is the preferred amount. You can also take power naps if you're unable to follow the eight hours of sleep rule.

Plus, if you get the right amount of sleep in your schedule, you'll be less grumpy when you wake up. For the ladies, you won't have to worry so much about breaking out anymore.

You'll be less stress and it'll be easier for you to put a smile on your face. You'll feel a lot healthier and you'll feel more active during the day.

Another benefit of sleeping is the fact that you can lose weight. I know, it sounds unbelievable right? Well, it's true. If you think that sleep can make you gain weight because you're not active then you're wrong.

When you sleep, your body starts to repair and recover itself. Now the reason why sleeping is able to help you lose weight is because when you're sleeping, the hormones that are used to help regulate your appetite isn't being disrupted by anything.

Basically, because you are not going to do anything for the rest of the night, your body is taking advantage of this process to do its own work.

In addition, sleep also helps boost your immune system and boost your energy, which makes you less vulnerable to diseases.

As an added bonus, your memory is also boosted when you are resting because your brain is processing the events of your day.

Chapter 4 – Happiness

A healthy person is a happy person. Likewise, a happy person is a healthy person. After getting rid of all those excessive pounds and knowing that you've reached the goal that you've set out for yourself, you'll find that you are a happier person than how you were before.

That is because you feel healthier, you feel better and more energized, and most importantly, you feel less stress than before.

If you were following the proper diet plan that you were supposed to then you'll be able to feel just like this.

You can even feel this way without having to finish the program. Just knowing that you are willing to take that extra step and make that change for yourself should be a good enough reason for you to be happy.

During the diet plan, staying positive is the key to success. No matter what happens, you have to remain positive and know that you can do it. It'll be easy for you to feel happy if you remain feeling positive.

There are many ways in order to be happy. If you're the type of person that is easily angered or just doesn't feel as happy as other people then this is a good section that you should read.

In life, there will be many, many, many events that will leave us unhappy. Sometimes, it's just what we see happening and other times, it will be caused by someone else.

However, do not let that discourage you. Don't always let yourself be easily affected by what goes on in your life. Always look on the bright side.

Appreciate and notice all the good little things that circulate you. For starters, it would help if you listed all the good things that happened to you for the day rather than the bad.

Be careful not to make any poor choices when you're angry because you might regret it later on in the long run.

There is always the option of giving. When we see that we can make someone happy then we ourselves will feel happy.

There are a lot of ways that you can give and the best way is to do community service. Everyone needs a helping hand so why not give a hand to your community.

Plus, doing community service will also keep you on your feet and off your couch.

Cleaning up your house is also another factor. Do you ever notice your mood suddenly changing the moment you arrive home?

That's probably because of the atmosphere of your house. Your house can either give off a positive atmosphere or a negative atmosphere.

I know that the moment I step into my house my positive mood is immediately gone. If you have this feeling then you need to find out the source of what is making you unhappy.

Most of the time it can be because your house is messy, or at least a certain part of your house is messy.

If that's the reason then you should cut back on your work out time and spend it by cleaning up the house.

It won't affect you much when you're cutting back your work out time by a little because you are still active as you're cleaning the house.

If you've been diagnosed with depression or any of the sorts then don't bother using anti-depressants because it can make you gain weight. If you don't want to feel depressed but don't know how then you should see a therapist.

Therapists are paid to help you over come any issues that you have regarding yourself. Follow through with that they tell you and take their advice because they are trained professionals who know that they are doing.

Health

I've said it before, happiness greatly contributes to health. Eating healthy, working out and sleeping are all important factors in being able to stay healthy. However, being happy is crucial because your mental health can also determine your physical health.

Negative thinking can bring you down in a lot of ways. You will be more vulnerable to stress and the higher the stress rate then the easier it will be for you to catch diseases.

The best way to improve your mental health is to always think positive.

I can't emphasize it anymore than I already have. Also, you might think that staying positive all the time is a hard thing to do.

It can be, especially if you're trying to force it out. Basically, all you have to do is relax. Don't over think and just do.

Every time you wake up, put an immediate smile on your face. You don't have to look at yourself in the mirror to give a big smile. As long as you don't start the day with a frown then you'll be on the safe side.

Don't forget to always keep yourself physically healthy. Take the tips that I've given you into consideration. Always drink water. Water is important.

When you are going on a diet, water is the best liquid that you can drink. It quenches your thirst and you won't gain any weight from it.

Of course, if you drink too much at once then you'll probably feel bloated for a while. Even so, it's best to drink about three to four bottles a day to keep yourself hydrated.

Water might be good but be careful not to drink too much in a day. Also, remember to exercise. Eat healthy food, about five to six servings per day. Keep a constant workout schedule and walk for about 30 minutes to an hour every day if you can.

Conclusion

Now that you've reached the end, you should have a clear idea as to what you should do and what you should not do.

Remember, when you decide in your mind that you want to start a diet program then you'll have to maintain that program for the rest of your life.

It might sound hectic to you now but after a few months of the same routine, it'll become a new habit that you've developed.

However, you should also be careful of the possible chances of you reverting back into your old habits.

It's going to be expected that you will start craving for certain foods about once or twice every month and that's perfectly normal.

It is human nature to crave and it's perfectly fine if you follow through with your cravings.

Keep in mind that you should come back on track as soon as possible. If you had some junk food for a snack before dinner then, for dinner, you should eat something healthy in order to balance out your calorie intake of the day.

Make sure that you don't ever skip a meal. Starving isn't the way to go if you want to succeed in losing weight.

Chances are, you will start to overeat in your next meal and you'll gain more weight because of the fat that your body stored from the lack of food.

Always be consistent with your exercise routine. If you're ever bored with exercising then you can always multitask and exercise while you are watching your favorite show. There's also the option of using the treadmill while reading a book.

If you go to the gym, you can always bring a workout partner with you. There are a few gyms out there that allow you to bring in a guest for free if you have a membership.

If you have a friend who has been trying to lose weight just think of it as an opportunity for the both of you to spend quality time together.

You'll feel less lonely knowing that you have a partner who is there for you every step of the way.

Don't forget to also consult to your family. Tell them what you are planning to do and have them support you through your program.

If anything, ask them to join you. It doesn't hurt to be healthy. Unfortunately, there are times when even your family members can't abide by your request.

The best support you can get is from your spouse because they are living with you. If you have kids then you don't have to worry because as a parent, you have absolute dominance over their lives until they become adults themselves.

If your parents live with you then you shouldn't have a hard time persuading them to follow through with your idea. I have to admit though, trying to persuade your spouse can become tricky.

It would be great they can follow through your idea and support you every step of the way. It's even better if they join you.

However, if your spouse mocks you or belittles you for any reason during your diet program then I think you should reevaluate your relationship with them.

Goals, goals, and goals. Always set a new goal for yourself every week and always remember to write down your goals so you won't forget.

You'll be more motivated to accomplish your goals if you see it written down rather than trying to keep it in your mind.

If anything, you can always resort to the pros and cons method. Basically, you'll be writing a list of how the program will benefit you and what would happen if you don't follow through with the program.

Once you're done, post that list at a place that will make you look at it everyday like the fridge. It'll be like your motivating factor during the program.

Lastly, remember to always stay positive and happy. Don't let your anger sour your mood for the rest of the day.

Know that you are always loved by the people around you and always spend some time giving love to others. Give at least eight hugs to the people around you.

You might not like hugs but they do make you feel better. I'm not saying that you should hug some random stranger that you've met on the streets, but you're free to do that if you want to.

Smile at everyone you see. Smiling is another form of greeting without the use of words. You don't have to give a big smile that makes you show your teeth. A simple smirk is perfectly fine. Anything that will stop you from frowning will give you a positive feeling for the rest of the day.

www.ingramcontent.com/pod-product-compliance
Lightning Source LLC
Chambersburg PA
CBHW050335290526
45785CB00006B/2505